DEFEATING DIABETES WITH EXPERT GUIDANCE

Ultimate Solution Handbook For Patients, Guardians Or Family To Understand, Manage, Treat, Prevent, Reverse Symptoms And Live Well

DR. POTTER WHITLEY

Copyright © 2023 by Dr. Potter Whitley

DISCLAIMER:

This book's contents are meant to be used solely for informative purposes. The information should not be used as a replacement for expert medical advice, diagnosis, or care.

The information contained in this book is accurate and reliable, having been verified by the author to the best of his ability. Nevertheless, the author disclaims all express and implied representations and warranties regarding the availability, correctness, appropriateness, completeness, and reliability of the material provided here. You bear full responsibility for any reliance you may have on such material.

For informational purposes, this book may make reference to or mention of certain people, things, websites, organizations, or other names. The author has no connection to, endorsement from, or recommendation for these organizations. The author's approval or validation is not implied by the inclusion of these references.

Any direct, indirect, incidental, special, or consequential damages resulting from using or not being able to use the material in this book are not covered by the author's liability policy. For medical advice and counsel particular to their circumstances, readers are advised to check with experienced healthcare specialists.

The content, materials, and information in this book are subject to change at any time without prior notice, at the author's discretion. The text may contain errors or omissions for which the author is not responsible.

By reading this book, you understand and accept the conditions of this disclaimer.

THE REASON BEHIND THIS BOOK

For those navigating the complex terrain of diabetes, "Defeating DIABETES With Expert Guidance" is an all-inclusive manual that provides a beacon of empowerment and information. The book begins with an introduction to diabetes, explaining its various forms, causes, and the significant effects it has on the body. This preliminary investigation is essential because it establishes the foundation for readers to understand the subtleties of the illness.

The book explores diagnosis and monitoring, going beyond simple recognition and giving readers the skills necessary to recognize symptoms and comprehend critical diagnostic testing. The need for consistent monitoring is emphasized in the book, which encourages a proactive approach to diabetes management and reinforces the idea that education is the first line of defense.

A crucial section that delves into the significance of diet in managing diabetes is devoted to expert insights into nutrition. This book becomes a reliable resource when it comes to making the kinds of food decisions that are fundamental to managing diabetes, from understanding the complexities of proteins, lipids, and carbs to providing helpful meal-planning tips.

The story moves smoothly into the topic of physical health, emphasizing the advantages of physical activity and outlining guidelines for safe and efficient practices. It is suggested that incorporating physical activity into daily living is a dynamic lifestyle adjustment that can spark good transformation, rather than merely following a prescribed regimen.

The detailed examination of drugs and therapies that follows offers a comprehensive grasp of diabetes drugs, insulin therapy, and new therapeutic modalities. With an emphasis on a comprehensive approach to diabetes care, the book blurs the lines between medication interventions and lifestyle changes.

Beyond the individual, the book looks at specific populations, providing specialized perspectives on how to manage diabetes in young people, expectant mothers, and the elderly. The emotional aspect of diabetes is also discussed, recognizing its influence and offering doable methods for maintaining emotional health, such as managing stress, creating support networks, and managing anxiety and depression associated with diabetes.

The book, crucially, turns its focus to prevention, explaining typical issues associated with diabetes and promoting routine examinations. The book transforms into a proactive manual for maintaining health and well-being by providing readers with techniques to avoid long-term issues.

Last but not least, "Defeating DIABETES With Expert Guidance" takes readers into the future by examining advancements in diabetes research and exciting new technology. The last chapters offer optimism by outlining a future free of diabetes and highlighting our shared path toward a more prosperous and healthy society.

TABLE OF CONTENT

CHAPTER ONE

THE NATURE OF DIABETES
Overview of Diabetes:

Diabetes is a chronic illness that affects millions of people worldwide. It is defined by high blood sugar levels that are brought on by either insufficient or inefficient insulin utilization by the body. The hormone insulin, which is generated by the pancreas, is essential for controlling blood sugar levels. Diabetes can cause major health issues if it is not properly managed. Three basic kinds of illness are commonly recognized: Type 1, Type 2, and Gestational Diabetes. Effective management and preventative actions depend on an understanding of the distinctions between these categories.

Diabetes comes in three forms: Type 1, Type 2, and Gestational Diabetes.

An autoimmune condition known as type 1 diabetes occurs when the immune system targets and kills the pancreatic beta cells that produce insulin. Insulin replacement therapy is required for the rest of one's life as a result of little to no insulin production. Insufficient insulin synthesis or an ineffective use of insulin by the body characterizes type 2 diabetes, which is the more common type. Its development is frequently influenced by genetics, lifestyle choices, and weight. Pregnancy can cause gestational diabetes, which affects blood sugar levels and needs to be closely monitored to avoid issues for the mother and the fetus. Different treatment strategies are required for each category due to their distinct problems.

Factors at Risk and Causes:

It is essential to comprehend the origins and risk factors of diabetes to prevent it and treat it early. Environmental causes and genetic predisposition play a part in the development of Type 1 diabetes, albeit the specific etiology is unknown. Obesity, sedentary lifestyles, and poor diets are all strongly associated with type 2 diabetes. There are genetic components as well; a family history of diabetes raises the risk. Hormonal changes during pregnancy have been linked to gestational diabetes. A history of gestational diabetes in prior pregnancies, age, and ethnicity can further increase the risk. Understanding these variables enables people to lead educated lives and enables medical professionals to put specific preventive measures in place.

Effects of Diabetes on the Human Body:

Diabetes affects many different organs and systems, which can result in acute and long-term problems. High blood sugar raises the risk of cardiovascular illnesses by causing blood vessel damage. Diabetes-related nerve degeneration, or diabetic neuropathy, can cause discomfort, numbness, and decreased sensation, especially in the limbs. Diabetic nephropathy, or kidney disease, is another dangerous consequence that can result in renal failure. Diabetes can lead to disorders like diabetic retinopathy, which is a primary cause of blindness, making the eyes particularly vulnerable. Moreover, diabetes weakens immunity, increasing a person's susceptibility to infections. Using routine monitoring, medication, lifestyle changes, and, in certain situations, surgical procedures, comprehensive care addresses these possible consequences. The complexity of the effects diabetes has on the body highlights the significance of proactive, all-encompassing approaches to diabetes care.

CHAPTER TWO

ASSESSMENT AND OBSERVATION
Diagnosing Symptoms of Diabetes:

An essential first step in the early detection and treatment of diabetes is identifying its symptoms. Diabetes is a chronic illness that arises from the body's inability to either use the insulin it does make properly or produce enough of it. It is simple to ignore the signs because they can be mild and appear gradually. Common signs and symptoms include weariness, impaired eyesight, increased thirst, frequent urination, unexplained weight loss, and sluggish wound healing.

Elevated blood sugar is one of the main symptoms. Various difficulties might arise when glucose accumulates in the bloodstream instead of being absorbed by cells. If someone has these symptoms, they should consult a doctor right away because treatment can slow the progression of the illness. In addition to being crucial for maintaining one's health, recognizing these indicators raises community awareness and motivates others to get help right away if they notice any possible symptoms.

Furthermore, it is crucial to comprehend how lifestyle factors relate to the symptoms of diabetes. Diabetes can occur as a result of poor food choices, sedentary lifestyles, and genetic predispositions. By being aware of these risk factors, people can take proactive steps to reduce their likelihood of acquiring diabetes and promote overall health.

Tests for Diagnosis: A1C, Blood Sugar, and More:

To effectively combat diabetes, an accurate diagnosis is essential. Determining the existence and severity of the ailment is mostly dependent on several diagnostic tests. Blood sugar levels give quick information on how well the body is utilizing glucose. Blood sugar levels can be determined by fasting plasma glucose testing, oral glucose tolerance tests, or random blood sugar tests. High values can be a sign of prediabetes or diabetes.

Another important diagnostic marker is glycated hemoglobin or A1C. This blood test calculates the blood sugar average for the previous two to three months.

It helps people with diabetes make treatment decisions and set goals by providing a more thorough understanding of long-term glucose management. To evaluate the efficacy of treatment regimens and make required modifications, these markers must be regularly monitored.

Tests for diagnosis also aid in the distinction between type 1 and type 2 diabetes. Though the underlying causes and therapies are different, they both include problems with insulin. Personalized care that targets the unique aspects of each patient's ailment is guaranteed by an accurate diagnosis.

The continued care of diseases is aided by diagnostic testing as well. Healthcare practitioners can use them to monitor patients' progress, spot problems, and modify treatment regimens as necessary.

It is imperative to take preventive measures to avoid long-term risks linked to uncontrolled diabetes, including kidney issues, nerve damage, and cardiovascular disease.

Consistent Monitoring Is Essential

A key component of effective diabetes control is routine monitoring. Once diagnosed, patients need to monitor their blood sugar levels, nutrition, exercise routine, and medication adherence regularly. Healthcare providers can modify treatment plans in real-time by using data from routine monitoring, which gives people the power to make educated decisions about their health.

Blood sugar monitoring gives important information on how drugs and lifestyle decisions affect blood sugar levels throughout the day. People can maintain optimal blood sugar control by spotting patterns and trends and making necessary adjustments.

This proactive strategy improves general health and enjoyment of life by preventing acute issues like hyper- or hypoglycemia.

Partnerships between patients and their healthcare providers are also promoted by adequate monitoring. Healthcare providers can provide tailored assistance and ensure treatment regimens stay effective by exchanging monitoring data and conducting regular check-ins. Regular monitoring also makes it easier to identify any departures from the target range early on, enabling timely action and reducing the likelihood of problems.

Routine physical examinations are crucial for managing diabetes-related problems, in addition to blood sugar monitoring. These could include renal function tests, cardiovascular evaluations, and eye exams to identify diabetic retinopathy. Timely intervention, which halts the advancement of these problems and promotes long-term health, is made possible by early detection of complications.

To sum up, identifying symptoms, getting tested for the disease, and adopting routine monitoring are essential parts of a thorough strategy to overcome diabetes. Together, these elements promote proactive management, tailored therapy, and early identification, which eventually improves the general health and well-being of people with diabetes.

CHAPTER THREE

NUTRITION EXPERT PERSPECTIVES
Diet's Function in Diabetes Management:

Diabetes must be managed holistically, with nutrition being the most important factor in regulating blood sugar levels. Preventing abrupt spikes and crashes in glucose intake and absorption is the main objective. A consistent release of energy and a slow rise in blood sugar levels are the results of eating a well-balanced diet high in whole foods.

It is important to pay attention to a food's glycemic index (GI). Low-glycemic items are recommended since they raise blood sugar levels more gradually and slowly, like whole grains, legumes, and non-starchy veggies. Limiting high-GI meals, such as processed grains and refined sugars, is advised since they can cause abrupt rises in blood sugar levels.

Another important factor is the distribution of macronutrients. Stable blood sugar levels can be attained with a diet that is well-balanced in terms of carbohydrates, proteins, and fats. Simple sugars should be avoided in favor of complex carbs, which are found in whole grains and veggies. Healthy fats, like those found in almonds and avocados, supply vital nutrients without having a major effect on blood sugar levels. Proteins aid in satiety and the maintenance of muscle development.

Furthermore, portion control is essential to balance calorie intake and avoid overindulging. Extreme blood sugar swings can be avoided with smaller, more frequent meals. It is vital to regularly check blood glucose levels to comprehend the effects of various foods on an individual and to make the appropriate dietary plan adjustments.

Understanding Fats, Proteins, and Carbohydrates:

A comprehensive knowledge of carbs, proteins, and lipids is essential for managing nutrition effectively in the setting of diabetes. Among macronutrients, carbohydrates are the main factor affecting blood sugar levels. Blood sugar rises as a result of their breakdown into glucose. All carbohydrates are not made equal, though. Whole grains and vegetables include complex carbs, which release energy gradually into the bloodstream and give long-lasting energy.

Proteins are necessary for several body processes, including the treatment of diabetes. They aid in satiety, which helps regulate hunger and stop overindulging. Furthermore, because proteins slow down the absorption of glucose, they help to stabilize blood sugar levels. It is advised to consume lean protein sources such as fish, poultry, tofu, and lentils.

For those with diabetes, a balanced diet must include healthy fats. Increased insulin sensitivity has been linked to monounsaturated and polyunsaturated fats, which are present in avocados, fatty fish, and olive oil. Conversely, as they may exacerbate insulin resistance, trans and saturated fats ought to be consumed in moderation.

It's critical to maintain this nutritional balance. No macronutrient should be severely restricted in a well-rounded diet; instead, a balance that meets each person's demands and aids in maintaining stable blood sugar levels should be the goal.

Planning Meals for People with Diabetes:

A systematic strategy for maintaining ideal blood sugar levels throughout the day is provided by meal planning, which is the cornerstone of diabetes treatment. Planning a well-thought-out meal plan entails taking into account the kinds and quantities of food eaten when to eat, and the general nutritional value.

Carbohydrate counting is a cornerstone of diabetic meal-planning strategies. People can better control their blood sugar levels when they are aware of the carbohydrate content of various foods. This entails choosing the appropriate kinds of carbs and paying attention to serving sizes.

Furthermore, diabetes meal planning frequently uses the idea of the plate method. Using this technique, a plate is visually divided into quarters for carbohydrates, quarters for lean protein, and half for non-starchy veggies. This straightforward yet efficient method supports blood sugar regulation by helping to create balanced meals.

Another crucial component of meal planning is timing. Blood sugar levels can be kept from fluctuating too much by eating at regular intervals throughout the day. Meal skipping can cause low blood sugar while eating too much can cause high blood sugar. Improved glycemic control is a result of quantity control and meal schedule consistency.

To achieve total nutritional demands, it is imperative to incorporate a variety of nutrient-dense foods. A wide range of vital vitamins and minerals are made sure to be consumed by people with diabetes through a varied and colorful assortment of fruits, vegetables, whole grains, lean proteins, and healthy fats. Personalized advice on creating a meal plan that suits one's tastes, way of life, and health objectives can be obtained by speaking with a licensed dietitian.

Superfoods together with Nutritional Approaches:

In the field of nutrition, the idea of "superfoods" has gained traction, and adding nutrient-dense superfoods to one's diet can have special advantages for those with diabetes. These foods are abundant in bioactive chemicals, vitamins, minerals, and antioxidants that support general health and may be especially beneficial for managing diabetes.

Because of their low glycemic index and high fiber content, berries including blueberries, strawberries, and raspberries are regarded as superfoods for diabetics. Berries include antioxidants that may help reduce oxidative stress related to diabetes.

Omega-3 fatty acids, which have anti-inflammatory qualities and may enhance insulin sensitivity, are abundant in fatty fish, such as salmon and mackerel. Fish consumption can be a beneficial nutritional approach for those who have diabetes.

Nuts and seeds—like almonds, chia, and flaxseeds—are nutrient-dense superfoods that offer a mix of fiber, protein, and healthy fats. In addition to providing a variety of vital nutrients, these foods aid in satiety and blood sugar regulation.

Rich in vitamins and minerals, leafy greens like kale, spinach, and collard greens are low in calories and carbs. In addition to promoting digestive health, its high fiber content may help regulate blood sugar.

Using particular nutritional approaches can improve diabetes management even more than adding superfoods. To promote a better relationship with food, mindful eating, for instance, advises paying attention to signals of hunger and fullness. A few helpful tactics for preserving steady blood sugar levels are meal planning, portion control, and awareness of emotional eating tendencies.

Frequently disregarded, hydration is essential for maintaining general health and managing diabetes. Maintaining proper digestion, avoiding dehydration, and managing weight can all be facilitated by drinking enough water.

It's critical to remember that there is no one-size-fits-all approach to diet, even while superfoods and other nutritional tactics might be helpful. Individuals can react differently to different meals, thus tailored diet regimens should take into account things like cultural norms, personal preferences, and any underlying medical issues. Personalized advice on optimizing nutrition for diabetes treatment can be obtained by consulting with healthcare professionals, such as registered dietitians.

CHAPTER FOUR

EXERCISE AND PHYSICAL ACTIVITY
Benefits of Physical Activity for Diabetes

For those who are controlling their diabetes, regular exercise has many advantages. Better blood sugar regulation is one of the main benefits. The hormone that controls blood sugar levels, insulin, is more sensitive to the body when it exercises. Because of their increased sensitivity, cells are more adept at absorbing glucose from the bloodstream, which lowers blood sugar levels overall.

Additionally, weight control is an essential component of managing diabetes, and exercise helps with this. Better insulin function and reduced insulin resistance are directly correlated with maintaining a healthy weight. Maintaining and reaching a healthy weight are facilitated by regular physical activity, which also increases metabolism, burns calories and builds lean muscle mass.

Moreover, cardiovascular health is improved by exercise, and this is especially crucial for people with diabetes. Diabetes is linked to a higher risk of heart disease, and regular exercise improves cholesterol levels, lowers blood pressure, and strengthens the heart. Thus, the chance of cardiovascular issues is decreased, which is good news for people with diabetes.

Furthermore, physical activity is essential for managing stress. Blood sugar levels can be negatively impacted by stress, and controlling diabetes can add to an individual's already high-stress levels. Exercise regularly releases endorphins, which improve mood, lower stress levels, and promote mental health in general. Exercise is a natural stress reliever.

In conclusion, exercise has several advantages for those with diabetes. Frequent physical activity is essential for managing diabetes well since it can lead to several benefits such as better blood sugar control, weight management, improved cardiovascular health, and reduced stress.

Establishing a Secure and Successful Workout Program:

For people with diabetes to maximize the health benefits of physical activity while lowering hazards, it is critical to establish a safe and efficient exercise regimen. It's important to speak with medical professionals before starting any fitness program to determine your demands, evaluate your current health, and rule out any potential contraindications.

A mix of strength training, flexibility training, and cardiovascular exercises should be part of the workout regimen. Exercises that increase cardiovascular health and promote blood sugar regulation include brisk walking, cycling, and swimming.

Exercises for developing muscle mass and increasing metabolism that involve resistance or weight-bearing activities can help with weight management and insulin sensitivity.

To avoid injuries and take into account each person's unique degree of fitness, it is imperative to begin cautiously and advance gradually. Understanding how the body reacts to physical activity and modifying the training regimen as needed depends on monitoring blood sugar levels before, during, and following exercise.

Selecting sustainable and pleasurable activities is equally vital. Maintaining a long-term fitness regimen requires consistency. Adherence to the program is more likely when enjoyable and fulfilling activities are found.

Incorporating safety precautions like wearing the right footwear, drinking plenty of water, and being aware of potential side effects like hypoglycemia before, during, and after exercise is also crucial.

Maintaining constant supervision and making necessary modifications to the workout program is ensured by regular contact with healthcare specialists.

Personalized planning, moderate progression, a variety of exercise modalities, and ongoing communication with healthcare providers are all necessary for a safe and successful exercise regimen that maximizes health benefits and minimizes hazards for people with diabetes.

Integrating Exercise into Everyday Life:

A realistic and long-term strategy for ensuring regular exercise for people with diabetes is to include physical activity in daily life. Making physical activity a fun and natural part of one's routine is the aim, as it promotes general health and well-being.

Finding times during the day to engage in accidental activity is one useful tactic. Taking the stairs instead of the elevator, parking further away from locations to promote walking, and fitting in quick bursts of exercise during work breaks are a few examples of basic behaviors that fall under this category. A rise in overall physical activity levels is a result of these modest but persistent efforts.

Choosing hobbies and pastimes that fit individual interests and preferences is another smart strategy. Participating in joyful activities increases the likelihood that people will persist with them over time, whether it be dancing, gardening, or leisure sports

. This benefits not just one's physical health but also one's mental and emotional wellness.

Adding a social element to physical activities with friends or family can also improve workout quality and provide extra motivation. Walking clubs and exercise courses are examples of group activities that build a supportive environment and a sense of community.

Technology can also be used to encourage regular exercise. People can easily stay motivated and accountable with the help of fitness monitors, smartphone applications, and internet resources that offer tools for tracking progress, setting goals, and accessing guided workouts.

In conclusion, integrating social support, using technology, choosing pleasurable activities, and making deliberate decisions are all important parts of integrating physical exercise into a person's everyday life for those with diabetes. To effectively manage diabetes, keeping an active lifestyle is crucial, and these techniques help to establish a sustainable and comprehensive approach to doing so.

CHAPTER FIVE

TREATMENT OPTIONS AND MEDICATION
An Overview of Drugs for Diabetes:

Diabetes must be managed with a multimodal strategy that frequently includes both medication and lifestyle changes. For diabetic treatment to be effective, it is essential to comprehend the different groups of drugs. Oral antidiabetic medications, which include DPP-4 inhibitors, sulfonylureas, and metformin, are one of the main groups. One first-line treatment that improves insulin sensitivity and lowers hepatic glucose production is metformin. While DPP-4 inhibitors control blood sugar by blocking the breakdown of incretin hormones, sulfonylureas promote the release of insulin from the pancreas.

The thiazolidinediones, which include pioglitazone, are another class of drugs that increase peripheral tissues' sensitivity to insulin. Similar to acarbose, alpha-glucosidase inhibitors moderate postprandial blood sugar rises by slowing down the intestinal absorption of carbohydrates. Furthermore, SGLT-2 inhibitors, such as empagliflozin, affect the kidneys, decreasing the reabsorption of glucose and increasing its excretion in urine.

GLP-1 receptor agonists are among the injectable drugs in addition to insulin. These medications, which include liraglutide, work by boosting the release of insulin and inhibiting the secretion of glucagon, just like incretin hormones do. They help postpone the emptying of the stomach, which aids in weight loss. Knowing the subtle differences between each class enables medical professionals to customize treatment regimens to meet the needs of each patient, taking into account costs, side effects, and comorbidities.

Types and Administration of Insulin Therapy:

Insulin is still the mainstay of diabetes care, particularly in more severe cases or when other drugs are not working well enough. Patients and healthcare practitioners need to understand the kinds and methods of administration. Lispro and other rapid-acting insulins work fast to reduce postprandial glucose rises. Regular insulin and other short-acting insulins have a somewhat delayed onset but last longer. Comparable in duration to NPH, intermediate-acting insulin is frequently used to regulate blood sugar levels in between meals.

The baseline level of insulin provided by long-acting insulin analogs, such as glargine and detemir, resembles the body's normal secretion. This contributes to steady blood sugar levels both during the day and at night. For many patients, combination insulin treatments that combine longer-acting insulin with short- or rapid-acting insulin present a more convenient choice.

Insulin pumps or subcutaneous injections are two ways in which insulin can be administered. A patient's lifestyle, preferences, and the requirement for accurate insulin delivery all play a role in the decision. Continuous glucose monitoring devices can be used in conjunction with insulin therapy to improve overall glycemic control by offering real-time data to inform insulin dosage adjustments.

New Technologies and Treatment Methods:

Novel therapy modalities and technologies have been introduced in the management of diabetes recently. A significant advancement is the introduction of continuous glucose monitoring (CGM) devices, which offer real-time information on blood sugar levels. These technologies enable diabetics and medical professionals to decide on insulin dosages and lifestyle modifications in a timely and knowledgeable manner.

Furthermore, studies are looking into the possibilities of artificial pancreas devices, or closed-loop insulin delivery systems. These devices lessen the strain of ongoing decision-making for diabetics by automating the supply of insulin based on real-time glucose measurement.

Regenerative medicine techniques are gaining popularity as an alternative to conventional drugs to regain pancreatic function. The ability to repair insulin-producing cells in the pancreas is being studied through stem cell therapy and beta-cell replacement therapy.

In conclusion, both diabetes patients and healthcare providers must stay current with these new treatment alternatives. It may be possible to improve glycemic control, lower complications, and raise the general quality of life for people with diabetes by implementing these technologies into comprehensive care programs.

CHAPTER SIX

DIABETES MANAGEMENT THROUGH LIFESTYLE CHANGES
Strategies for Stress Management:

Because stress causes the release of stress hormones like cortisol and adrenaline, which raise blood sugar levels, stress is a ubiquitous factor that can have a substantial impact on managing diabetes. People with diabetes must put appropriate stress management strategies into practice. One strategy is mindfulness meditation, which promotes developing awareness without passing judgment and remaining in the present moment. Regular mindfulness meditation has been demonstrated in studies to reduce stress and enhance glycemic control. Furthermore, useful techniques for reducing stress include yoga and deep breathing exercises. Physical activity can help reduce stress and improve general well-being. Examples of this include walking, jogging, and playing sports.

Stress management can be further aided by incorporating relaxation techniques like progressive muscle relaxation or biofeedback. People can identify and treat physical signs of stress, such as tense muscles, with the help of these techniques. Individuals can get coping mechanisms and emotional support by creating a support network and getting professional assistance through counseling or therapy. People with diabetes can effectively manage their blood sugar levels and improve their overall quality of life by adopting a multimodal approach to stress management.

Sleep Quality and Its Effect on Blood Sugar:

Sleep and diabetes have a complex relationship, and blood sugar management is greatly influenced by the quantity and quality of sleep. Sleep deprivation, whether whole or partial, can upset the hormonal equilibrium and cause insulin resistance and elevated blood sugar. A regular sleep schedule that includes a set bedtime and wake-up time helps improve blood sugar regulation. To encourage good sleep, it's essential to follow sleep hygiene guidelines including making a cozy sleeping environment and avoiding stimulants just before bed.

Studies show that decreased glucose metabolism may occur in diabetics who suffer from sleep deprivation. This highlights the need to treat sleep disorders, including sleep apnea, which is common among people with diabetes. Improved glycemic control has been linked to continuous positive airway pressure (CPAP) therapy, a standard treatment for sleep apnea. Stressing the significance of sleep as a cornerstone of diabetes care encourages people to modify their lifestyles in ways that improve their blood sugar control and quality of sleep.

The Link Between Diabetes and Quitting Smoking:

One modifiable risk factor that greatly aggravates the effects of diabetes is smoking. Cardiovascular disorders are already a big worry for people with diabetes who smoke. Smokers are more likely to develop these conditions. Giving up smoking is a crucial component of managing diabetes since it lowers the risk of cardiovascular problems and enhances general health outcomes.

Tobacco smoke contains noxious compounds that can increase inflammation and directly impact insulin sensitivity, leading to insulin resistance. Improved insulin sensitivity and improved blood sugar regulation have been linked to quitting smoking. It also reduces the chance of getting diabetic nephropathy and peripheral vascular disease, two other problems linked to the illness.

A combination of behavioral therapies, psychotherapy, and medicine is used to support individuals in their journey to stop smoking. Healthcare professionals can assist patients in making major progress toward improved general health and lessen the influence of this modifiable risk factor on their diabetes prognosis by emphasizing smoking cessation as a key component of diabetes care.

CHAPTER SEVEN

DIABETES IN SPECIAL POPULATIONS
Diabetes and Children:

Children with diabetes present particular difficulties that call for particular attention and treatment. The most prevalent type of diabetes in children is called type 1, in which the immune system unintentionally targets and kills the pancreatic cells that produce insulin. Maintaining a healthy lifestyle, monitoring blood glucose levels, and administering insulin to children with diabetes requires a careful balance. To ensure appropriate management, parents, caregivers, and healthcare professionals must collaborate, as children may not completely understand the significance of their condition.

When navigating school, peer interactions, and extracurricular activities, children with diabetes frequently have social and emotional difficulties. Building a supportive environment for students with diabetes requires educating instructors, classmates, and friends about the disease. Including kids in their treatment and emphasizing the value of following prescription instructions and adopting healthy behaviors also gives them the confidence to actively manage their illness.

To effectively manage diabetes in children, nutrition is essential. Their daily routine starts to include things like keeping an eye on their blood sugar levels, eating regular meals, and balancing their consumption of carbohydrates. To create customized treatment regimens, families, nutritionists, and healthcare professionals must work together. The care of diabetes in children has also been enhanced by ongoing technology breakthroughs, such as continuous glucose monitoring systems, which offer real-time data for fast insulin dosage adjustments.

Diabetes is a Mother-to-Be:

Pregnancy can cause gestational diabetes, a kind of disease that needs to be closely monitored because it can affect both the mother and the fetus. Blood sugar levels rise as a result of the body's inability to manufacture enough insulin to satisfy the increasing demands of pregnancy. Pregnancy-related diabetes management calls for a multidisciplinary strategy that includes close observation and coordination between endocrinologists, obstetricians, and diabetes educators.

Risks associated with uncontrolled gestational diabetes include hypertension, preterm birth, and an increased chance of cesarean delivery. As a result, regular testing to check blood glucose levels becomes essential for customizing treatment regimens. The cornerstones of controlling gestational diabetes are dietary changes and physical activity, with an emphasis on keeping blood sugar levels within advised ranges.

Effective blood glucose control may require medical interventions like insulin therapy or oral medicines. Careful thought must be given to weighing the advantages of medicine against any possible hazards to the developing fetus. Frequent prenatal exams, fetal monitoring, and ultrasounds become crucial parts of diabetes management during pregnancy to guarantee mother and child health.

Taking Care of Seniors with Diabetes:

Diabetes management presents unique obstacles for the senior population, which are frequently exacerbated by age-related health problems and possible cognitive loss. An individualized strategy that takes functional limits, drug interactions, and comorbidities into account is needed for the management of diabetes in the elderly. To guarantee the best possible care, close coordination between medical professionals, caregivers, and the old person is essential.

An essential component of diabetes care for the elderly is medication control. Due to the prevalence of polypharmacy in older persons, a thorough medication assessment is necessary to prevent negative interactions and side effects. Reminders and the simplification of prescription schedules can improve adherence.

Nutrition and exercise are important factors in the management of diabetes in the elderly. Exercise regimens should be adjusted to account for mobility problems, and a healthy diet should be the main priority. It is more crucial than ever to regularly check blood glucose levels because swings might be modest and go unrecognized.

In the senior population, routine testing for consequences such as neuropathy, retinopathy, and cardiovascular disease is crucial. The general state of health and quality of life are enhanced by preventive measures, early identification, and timely intervention. Including caregivers in the treatment plan and offering assistance with everyday diabetes care activities become essential components of ensuring optimal outcomes for older adults with diabetes, as cognitive ability may diminish with age.

CHAPTER EIGHT

DIABETES AND EMOTIONAL HEALTH
Taking Care of Diabetes's Emotional Impact:

People who have diabetes may experience severe emotional effects. A diabetes diagnosis can cause a person to experience a wide range of emotions, such as grief, anxiety, and dread. It can be depressing to realize that major lifestyle adjustments may be necessary and that issues may arise. It is essential to address the emotional impact on general well-being.

Developing self-awareness is one important component. Emotional management begins with recognizing and acknowledging one's feelings. Mental health is just as important as physical health when managing diabetes.

Getting professional assistance, like therapy or counseling, can provide people with the skills they need to deal with the emotional difficulties brought on by diabetes. Within the diabetes community, it is imperative to de-stigmatize obtaining mental health support.

Education also has a major impact. Giving people thorough knowledge about diabetes and how it affects their emotions can enable them to take charge of their mental health.

Comprehending the correlation between stress and blood sugar levels, for instance, empowers people to make knowledgeable decisions regarding stress mitigation.

Furthermore, it is imperative to foster a positive outlook. Resilience can be developed by encouraging people to concentrate on the things they can control rather than the things they cannot. A sense of community can be fostered through forums and group activities where people can share their experiences, which helps lessen the isolation that is frequently linked to long-term illnesses.

Creating a strong support network is crucial for people with diabetes. Family, friends, medical experts, and even internet communities can provide a support system. These networks are essential for offering encouragement, practical help, and emotional support.

Involvement from the family is especially important. Teaching family members about diabetes promotes empathy and understanding. This makes it possible for them to offer the required assistance, such as dietary modifications and psychological support. A cooperative approach to managing diabetes is established when there is clear communication within the family.

Healthcare providers are essential components of the support network. Establishing routine check-ins, being transparent about difficulties, and working together to make decisions all improve the patient-provider connection.

Diabetes management is a team effort, and a thorough and individualized strategy is ensured by solid cooperation with healthcare providers.

A distinct kind of help is provided by online forums and support groups. Developing relationships with those who are experiencing comparable circumstances can help people feel less alone. These sites offer a forum for the exchange of advice, success stories, and coping mechanisms. But it's important to make sure that the data from these sources correspond with expert medical advice.

Handling Depression and Stress Associated with Diabetes:

People with diabetes frequently experience emotional difficulties such as stress and depression. Stress levels might be increased by the demands of managing the condition daily as well as worries about possible complications. To preserve mental health, coping mechanisms are essential.

Techniques for stress management are one useful strategy. These can include regular physical activity, deep breathing techniques, and mindfulness meditation. Taking part in enjoyable and soothing activities can help you feel less stressed. It's critical to customize these tactics to each person's preferences to make sure they are long-term viable.

Early treatments for depression require an understanding of its symptoms. If someone with diabetes feels depressed, despondent, or loses interest in activities regularly, they should be encouraged to get professional assistance. Diabetes self-care can be impacted by depression, so it's critical to treat mental health issues in addition to physical ones.

It is crucial to include mental health in the overall strategy for managing diabetes. Regular check-ups for medical care should include routine evaluations for emotional well-being. By taking a proactive stance, mental health issues can be identified early and treated, preventing them from getting worse.

Additionally, developing resilience is essential to managing the stress and despair brought on by diabetes. Creating flexible coping strategies, keeping an optimistic attitude, and embracing a sense of purpose are all part of building resilience. Diabetes care programs should incorporate education on resilience-building techniques to help people manage the emotional challenges of having diabetes.

CHAPTER NINE

AVOIDING ADVERSE EVENTS
Common Diabetes Complications:

Chronic metabolic diseases like diabetes can cause a wide range of problems that have a major negative influence on a person's health and quality of life. Heart-related conditions are among the most common consequences. A significant risk factor for strokes, heart attacks, and other cardiovascular problems is diabetes. High blood sugar levels cause plaque to build up in the arteries, which causes atherosclerosis and makes people more vulnerable to heart-related issues.

Diabetic neuropathy is another serious complication that can cause numbness, tingling, and pain in the extremities. It damages the nerves. This might eventually lead to more serious issues including infections and foot ulcers, which can seriously jeopardize one's ability to move around and general well-being. Diabetic nephropathy is another condition where kidney function is compromised by diabetes. As the kidneys' capacity to remove waste from the blood decreases, toxins build up and the risk of renal failure rises.

Diabetes is also linked to vision impairment and blindness, mainly as a result of diabetic retinopathy. If treatment is not received, this disorder affects the blood vessels in the retina, impairing vision and perhaps resulting in blindness.

Furthermore, diabetes weakens the immune system, increasing a person's susceptibility to infections. Slow healing and chronic wounds are common, and this increases the risk of infections, which can be difficult to manage.

Patients with diabetes and their healthcare providers must recognize and comprehend these problems. Comprehensive health assessments and routine blood pressure, cholesterol, and blood glucose monitoring can aid in the early detection and treatment of these issues, ultimately halting their progression.

The Value of Routine Checkups

Frequent examinations are essential for managing diabetes since they work as a proactive measure to successfully monitor and control the illness. A thorough assessment of numerous health markers, such as blood pressure, cholesterol, blood glucose, and renal function, is part of these check-ups.

To maintain ideal glycemic control, blood glucose levels must be regularly monitored. It makes it possible for medical professionals to modify medicine, food, and lifestyle choices as needed, avoiding abrupt changes in blood sugar levels that may lead to issues. As hypertension is a major cause of cardiovascular problems and a prevalent coexisting illness in people with diabetes, routine blood pressure monitoring is equally crucial.

Because of the strong correlation between cardiovascular health and cholesterol levels, lipid profiles can be evaluated and managed with routine checkups. An increased risk of heart attacks and strokes can result from atherosclerosis, which is exacerbated by abnormal cholesterol levels. Tests for kidney function are essential for spotting the early warning signs of diabetic nephropathy so that prompt therapies can stop the condition from getting worse.

Regular check-ups give medical professionals the chance to evaluate general health, address potential risk factors, and provide advice on lifestyle improvements in addition to these physiological indicators. People with diabetes can control their condition more actively by learning about healthy eating, regular exercise, and stress reduction. This will improve their general health and lower their risk of complications.

Regular follow-ups with medical staff build a cooperative connection that encourages candid dialogue and trust. The diabetes management plan can be promptly adjusted thanks to this continuous communication, which takes into account each person's unique response and evolving health. All things considered, routine examinations are essential to the prevention and early identification of complications associated with diabetes, enabling people to live longer, healthier lives.

Techniques for Avoiding Prolonged Issues:

Diabetes's long-term consequences can be avoided with a multimodal strategy that takes into account several facets of lifestyle and health. Keeping your blood sugar levels under ideal control with a combination of medicine, food, and regular exercise is one of the key tactics. Regular blood glucose monitoring lowers the risk of problems by assisting patients and healthcare professionals in making educated decisions to maintain blood sugar within target ranges.

Maintaining a healthy lifestyle is essential to avoiding long-term issues. Diabetes sufferers should prioritize a balanced diet full of whole grains, fruits, vegetables, lean meats, and healthy fats because nutrition is so important. Better blood sugar regulation is facilitated by mindful eating, portion control, and carbohydrate intake monitoring. Reducing alcohol intake and quitting smoking are also crucial lifestyle choices that promote general health.

A key component of managing diabetes and preventing complications is regular physical activity. Exercise helps control weight, raises insulin sensitivity, and lowers blood sugar. Additionally, it improves cardiovascular health by lowering the risk of problems associated with the heart. Depending on their fitness levels and medical conditions, people with diabetes should perform a mix of aerobic, strength, and flexibility exercises.

Controlling blood pressure and cholesterol levels is essential to preventing complications. When prescribed, medications must be taken exactly as instructed. In addition, lifestyle changes including frequent exercise and a low-sodium diet can support pharmaceutical therapies. Scheduling routine examinations with medical professionals is essential for keeping an eye on these indicators and modifying treatment regimens as necessary.

Another crucial tactic is educating people with diabetes about the value of taking care of their feet. Diabetes-related complications like diabetic neuropathy and foot ulcers can be avoided with routine foot examinations, good hygiene, and quick attention to any indications of injury or infection.

Furthermore, it's important to pay attention to mental health. Emotional health and stress reduction are essential components of a comprehensive diabetes care plan. Prolonged stress can raise blood sugar levels, therefore methods of reducing stress including mindfulness, meditation, and counseling are important aids in preventing complications.

In conclusion, preventing long-term problems from diabetes necessitates a customized, all-encompassing strategy that takes into account other lifestyle factors in addition to glycemic management. Developing healthy behaviors, educating people, and preserving a cooperative connection between patients and medical professionals are all essential steps in the process of avoiding and treating issues associated with diabetes.

CHAPTER TEN

RESEARCH AND TRENDS IN DIABETES IN THE FUTURE
Novel Approaches to Diabetes Research:

Recent years have seen several ground-breaking discoveries in the field of diabetes research that have great potential to transform our understanding and treatment of this chronic illness. The field of genetic research has made significant strides in revealing the complex interactions between hereditary and environmental factors that contribute to the vulnerability to diabetes. Personalized therapy is now possible because of the discovery of particular genetic markers linked to diabetes risk, which allows for customized interventions and therapies.

Furthermore, the science of precision medicine has made significant strides, with scientists using cutting-edge tools like CRISPR-Cas9 to modify genes linked to diabetes. This holds promise for gene therapies that could target the underlying causes of the disease in addition to offering insights into the genetic basis of diabetes. Diabetes research has been further accelerated by the development of big data analytics and artificial intelligence, which have made it easier to analyze enormous datasets to find trends, anticipate complications, and improve treatment approaches.

The creation of wearables and smart gadgets that allow for continuous blood glucose monitoring represents another frontier in innovation. These gadgets improve the ability to gather data in real-time and provide people with diabetes the ability to make knowledgeable decisions about their course of care and lifestyle. By combining these technologies with telemedicine platforms, it is now possible to monitor patients remotely, which encourages a proactive approach to managing diabetes.

Moreover, research on the relationship between diabetes and the gut microbiota has become increasingly interesting. Studies reveal that the makeup of gut bacteria affects metabolic functions, and modifying the microbiome may have therapeutic benefits. An exciting new area of diabetes research is the potential beneficial effects of probiotics and microbiome-modulating therapies on glucose metabolism.

In summary, advances in diabetes research span a wide range of disciplines, including precision medicine, genetics, and the incorporation of cutting-edge technologies. These advancements not only broaden our knowledge of the condition but also present viable paths toward patient-centered, tailored, and more efficient diabetes care.

Innovative Technologies and Treatments:

The growing body of promising technologies and therapeutics targeted at better controlling and maybe preventing diabetes advances along with our understanding of the condition. One noteworthy breakthrough is the introduction of closed-loop insulin administration devices, sometimes known as "artificial pancreas." These systems use automated insulin delivery in conjunction with continuous glucose monitoring (CGM) to keep blood glucose levels within a desired range. In terms of improving glycemic control and lessening the load on those who have diabetes, this is a major advancement.

Furthermore, the area of regenerative medicine has demonstrated promise about diabetes. The goal of stem cell therapies and tissue engineering methods is to repair beta cells that produce insulin, which addresses the fundamental shortfall associated with type 1 diabetes.

There is hope for a treatment for diabetes thanks to ongoing clinical trials investigating the transplantation of functioning pancreatic cells and the use of stem cells to create cells that secrete insulin.

Notable progress has also been made in drug therapy, with an emphasis on new drugs that target several pathways involved in glucose metabolism. Modern medication classes like SGLT-2 inhibitors and GLP-1 receptor agonists have shown promise in enhancing glycemic control and lowering cardiovascular risk, in addition to conventional insulin and oral hypoglycemic medications.

Furthermore, diabetes treatment has changed as a result of the incorporation of mobile applications and digital health solutions.

Through apps that support medication adherence, lifestyle changes, and self-monitoring, people can take an active role in their care. Healthcare professionals can now remotely monitor patients thanks to this technology, providing prompt interventions and individualized advice.

In summary, the field of prospective diabetic treatments and technology is broad and dynamic. These technological advancements, which range from digital health tools to regenerative medicine and artificial pancreas systems, have the potential to change the way diabetes is treated and offer more efficient and user-friendly options.

The Path Ahead: Toward a Future Free of Diabetes:

The goal of eradicating diabetes calls for a thorough, multifaceted strategy that goes beyond the boundaries of care and therapy. With a rising focus on lifestyle treatments and population-wide measures to decrease diabetes risk factors, prevention emerges as a critical focal area. To achieve this, public health programs that encourage improved eating habits, more exercise, and awareness campaigns are essential.

The idea of metabolic health is one topic to research in the race to end diabetes. It may be possible to avoid the development of diabetes and its complications by changing the paradigm from treating diabetes alone to addressing more general metabolic health concerns. Insulin resistance, metabolic syndrome, and obesity-related strategies can all work together to lessen the overall burden of diabetes.

In addition, social determinants of health and community-based interventions are becoming more and more well-known.

The significance of comprehensive approaches is highlighted by the realization that diabetes risk is influenced by environmental variables, healthcare accessibility, and socioeconomic factors. To promote healthy living and aid in the prevention of diabetes, communities must work together with legislators, healthcare professionals, and community leaders.

Research-wise, a promising area of focus is the ongoing investigation of preventive vaccinations against particular forms of diabetes, especially type 1 diabetes. Preventive measures could be made possible by comprehending the autoimmune mechanisms that cause beta-cell death and creating therapies to stop or modify these processes.

Furthermore, promoting global cooperation and knowledge exchange is essential for eradicating diabetes in the future. Due to the diabetes epidemic's global scope, cooperation in research, policy creation, and healthcare delivery is required. By ensuring that innovations reach people in a variety of socio-cultural situations, collaborative projects can expedite the translation of research findings into workable solutions.

In summary, achieving a diabetes-free future will require a multimodal strategy that includes community-based interventions, preventive, holistic healthcare approaches, and international cooperation. Society can strive towards a future in which the prevalence of diabetes is drastically decreased, if not completely abolished, by addressing the underlying causes, risk factors, and social determinants of the disease.